DR. SEBI CURE FOR ALL DISEASES

The Bit by Bit Guide on Effective Natural Ways to Treat and Get Rid of Arthritis, Tinnitus, Psoriasis, Impotence, Stds, Pcos, Herpes, Diabetes, Cancer and Glaucoma

Justin Wescott
Copyright@2024

TABLE OF CONTENT
CHAPTER 1 2
   INTRODUCTION 2
CHAPTER 2 5
   What are the different causes of Diseases and Illnesses 5
CHAPTER 3 12
   DR SEBI CURE FOR TERRIBLE DISEASES 12
THE END 53

CHAPTER 1

INTRODUCTION

The plant-based diet embodies an alkaline approach, crafted to support the body's natural ability to heal by integrating a mindful eating plan with the use of supplements.

The designer known as Dr. Sebi, originally named Alfredo Darrington Bowman, was born in 1933 in Honduras.

The dietary approach advocates for a strict vegan lifestyle, rooted in the belief that all ailments stem from a specific dysfunction within the body's mucus membranes. Bowman suggested that fostering an alkaline environment can lead to the eradication of diseases.

Bowman's diet includes a Nutritional Guide that outlines a specific list of permissible foods, along with additional guidelines to follow.

Guidelines for the dietary approach (according to Bowman):

1. If the food isn't included in his Nutritional Guide, it is best to avoid it.
2. Consume one gallon of pure spring water daily.

3. Any products from Dr. Sebi should be consumed an hour prior to taking any medications.

4. All Dr. Sebi products can be combined without any concerns of interaction.

5. Following the Nutritional Guide closely, along with the recommended supplemental products, yields the most effective outcomes for reversing disease.

6. Sebi suggests that using the microwave will kill your food, so it's best to steer clear of it.

An alkaline diet focuses on the idea of balancing your body's pH through the selection of your food choices. The foods we consume can create metabolic waste, which may have a pH that ranges from alkaline to acidic.

The human body maintains various pH levels across different regions to facilitate unique physiological processes, with organs such as the stomach exhibiting higher acidity, while blood tends to be more alkaline. The balance of pH in different organs and fluids is carefully maintained.

Our body possesses remarkable systems for maintaining a harmonious balance, utilizing the lungs, kidneys, and various buffers to manage acidity and alkalinity through intricate processes of excretion and reabsorption. The food and fluids we consume have a direct influence on one of our bodily products: urine. This illustrates a process by which the kidneys help regulate the acidity and alkalinity of the blood.

CHAPTER 2

What are the different causes of Diseases and Illnesses

Causes of Illnesses
Illness encompasses a wide range of conditions that reflect an imbalance in the mind, body, and, to some degree, spirit. It is the overall sensation of discomfort or malaise, regardless of one's perception of being healthy.

Many individuals often conflate disease and illness, yet there are nuanced differences between the two. An ailment is the disturbance of a particular organ or the whole body caused by detrimental microorganisms like bacteria or viruses, physical harm, chemical imbalances, exposure to harmful substances, and the formation of underdeveloped cells. Some examples of ailments include cancer, fractures, diabetes, cirrhosis, and psoriasis, among others. Similar considerations apply to mental health challenges like bipolar disorder, clinical depression, and schizophrenia.

Illness, in contrast, reflects the body's response to disease. It signifies exhaustion, elevated temperature, diminished muscle strength, or unclear eyesight, along with irregular blood pressure and a quickened heartbeat. It is important to recognize that feeling unwell or experiencing discomfort can happen even in the absence of a specific illness.

Another difference between a disease and an illness lies in its specificity. An illness is determined by particular elements or standards that healthcare professionals assess when an individual seeks evaluation at a clinic or hospital. A condition, on the other hand, can encompass any ailment. Additionally, since it is primarily an experience, it may vary from one individual to another.

Factors Contributing to the Condition

A variety of factors can contribute to the onset of an illness, including the following:

The occurrence of ailments – Typically, health issues arise due to an underlying condition within the body. The body is inherently equipped to respond to any irregularity or danger, be it a bacterium, virus, or an overproduction of immature cells. However, this response can lead to feelings of discomfort in an individual. An excellent illustration is allergies. Allergies arise when the body's defense mechanism responds to perceived threats, leading to the release of histamines as part of its protective efforts. However, an individual might carry an illness yet still experience a sense of well-being. Conditions like HIV, AIDS, and cancer may take a considerable amount of time, sometimes months or years, before they manifest and affect a person's well-being.

Hypochondriasis – This condition explains why individuals may experience sensations of illness even in the absence of any actual disease. This condition pertains to an unusual or significant level of anxiety regarding the possibility of having an illness. A slight variation in body temperature might be perceived by someone overly concerned about their health as a fever or an indication of a grave illness such as cancer. The Internet today amplifies concerns about health and wellness. Individuals can now effortlessly explore their symptoms or engage in self-assessment.

Stress is an inherent reaction of the body to a stimulus. The body is inherently equipped to respond to stressful situations with a natural instinct for survival, activating either a fight or flight response. Regardless of the situation, it may elevate the heart rate and blood pressure, potentially resulting in the release of a hormone known as cortisol, which can contribute to illness when stress persists over time.

Malnutrition – The body is a complex system that requires a variety of enzymes, vitamins, minerals, and other macro and micronutrients to operate at its best. Over time, a lack of these essential elements can lead to feelings of unwellness in the body.

In holistic practices, like CTM (Chinese traditional medicine), an ailment can arise from an obstruction in the flow of vital energy (qi).
Essential Indicators

Health challenges can present with unclear signs, including:

Lightheadedness
Loose stools
Discomfort in the chest (or any form of discomfort)
Unease
Exhaustion
Irregular heart rhythm and fluctuating blood pressure
Clouded sight
Shaking

These symptoms could indicate various types of ailments, or they might have been amplified based on an individual's perception of their health condition.

Causes of Diseases
Microorganisms. These single-celled entities can lead to various ailments, including strep throat, urinary tract infections, and tuberculosis.
Illnesses. Even tinier than bacteria, these microscopic entities lead to a wide array of illnesses — from the familiar cold to more serious conditions like AIDS.
Fungi. Numerous skin conditions, including ringworm and athlete's foot, stem from fungal infections. Various fungi have the potential to invade your lungs or nervous system.

Unwanted invaders. Various parasites can be passed on to humans through the feces of animals.
Personal connection

One of the simplest ways to contract various infectious diseases is through contact with an infected person or animal. Three ways that illnesses can be transmitted through direct contact are:

Individual to individual. Infectious diseases often spread through the direct transfer of bacteria, viruses, or other germs between individuals. This can happen when a person carrying the bacterium or virus makes contact, shares a kiss, or coughs or sneezes near someone who is not infected.

These microorganisms can also be transmitted through the sharing of bodily fluids during intimate interactions. The individual who transmits the germ might not exhibit any signs of illness, yet could merely be a carrier.

Connection between creature and human. Getting bitten or scratched by an animal that carries an infection — even one you consider a pet — can lead to illness and, in severe cases, may result in death. Dealing with animal waste can pose risks as well. For instance, handling your cat's litter box can lead to a toxoplasmosis infection.

Guardian to the little one within. A woman expecting a child might transmit germs that lead to infectious diseases to her developing baby. Certain germs have the ability to traverse the placenta. Microorganisms present in the vaginal area can be passed on to the baby during the birthing process.

Subtle connection

Pathogens can also be transmitted through indirect contact.

When you come into contact with a doorknob that has been touched by someone suffering from the flu or a cold, you may acquire the germs they left behind.

Bug bites

Certain microorganisms depend on insect carriers — like mosquitoes, fleas, lice, or ticks — to transfer between hosts. These carriers are referred to as vectors. Insects like mosquitoes can transmit harmful diseases such as malaria or West Nile virus, while deer ticks may harbor the bacteria responsible for Lyme disease.

Contamination of food
Another way that harmful germs can enter your body is through food and water that are not clean. This method of spreading enables pathogens to reach numerous individuals from one origin. E. coli is a type of bacterium that can be found in or on specific foods, including undercooked hamburger and unpasteurized fruit juice.

CHAPTER 3

DR SEBI CURE FOR TERRIBLE DISEASES

Arthritis
Numerous plants can assist in alleviating the discomfort associated with arthritis. Herbs that reduce inflammation are particularly beneficial for connective tissues, while those that modulate the immune system can support conditions related to autoimmune arthritis. Additionally, herbs rich in minerals can aid in the repair and regeneration of joints and connective tissues. Incorporating more herbs that promote digestive wellness, enhance liver function, and aid in cleansing can be quite beneficial. Herbs abundant in bioflavonoids offer support for collagen protection. Discover some of the most powerful herbs for alleviating arthritis and learn how to incorporate them into your routine.

Ginger Root

Ginger is a root often utilized in culinary practices and serves as a remedy for a range of health issues, including arthritis. This substance is rich in compounds that are recognized for their ability to reduce inflammation and alleviate discomfort.

Ginger is wonderful for the digestive system, promoting smooth movement and supplying prebiotic material to the beneficial bacteria in your gut. Since a significant portion of our immune function relies on the health of our digestive system, maintaining its optimal performance is essential.

Ginger offers a variety of ways to enjoy its benefits, such as in a soothing cup of tea. For a soothing ginger tea, take fresh ginger and either grate or slice about 1 tablespoon. If using dried ginger, 1 teaspoon will do. Allow it to steep in hot water for 5-7 minutes to extract its natural essence. Consider enhancing the flavor with a touch of honey and a squeeze of lemon. Consuming ginger tea on a regular basis may support the reduction of inflammation and provide relief from joint discomfort. One of the most delightful ways to enjoy ginger is by incorporating it into a soothing chai tea latte.

Golden Spice

Turmeric is a spice that has been cherished in Indian cuisine and has a long-standing history in traditional healing practices. This compound contains curcumin, known for its soothing and protective qualities against inflammation and oxidative stress. Arthritis represents a condition influenced by oxidative stress, making the role of antioxidants vital in these situations. Turmeric has the potential to alleviate inflammation in connective tissues, offer pain relief, and slow down the progression of conditions like osteoarthritis and autoimmune diseases. Turmeric is wonderful for supporting the liver, which serves as our body's natural filtration system. When our liver functions optimally, our digestive system also thrives, and as mentioned earlier, there is a connection between digestion and arthritis.

Research indicates that curcumin may assist in decreasing inflammation within the body and easing joint discomfort. Consider incorporating a touch of black pepper to enhance the body's ability to absorb curcumin effectively. Or savor this perfectly blended Golden Turmeric Spice tea as a delightful Golden Latte.

Boswellia, also known as Indian Frankincense
Boswellia, often referred to as Indian frankincense, is a resin derived from the Boswellia serrata tree. This remedy has a long history in traditional Indian medicine, where it has been utilized for

centuries to address inflammatory conditions.

Boswellia is rich in compounds known as boswellic acids, celebrated for their ability to reduce inflammation. Research indicates that Boswellia may assist in diminishing inflammation within the body and easing discomfort in the joints. Boswellia can be enjoyed as a soothing tea or taken in the form of a capsule or tincture for its beneficial properties. We choose to utilize this herb in a tincture form, as it is derived from a resin and does not produce the most pleasant tasting tea.

Devil's Claw

Devil's claw, originating from Southern Africa, has a long history of use in addressing various health issues, including arthritis. Devil's claw is known for its iridoid glycosides, which are recognized for their ability to reduce inflammation and alleviate pain.

To prepare a soothing tea from devil's claw, simply steep a teaspoon of the dried root in a cup of hot water for 5-7 minutes.

Nettle Infusion

Nettle tea has been cherished for generations as a soothing solution for joint discomfort and swelling. Nettle is abundant in vitamins and minerals such as calcium, magnesium, and iron, and it has demonstrated a strong anti-inflammatory effect on the body. Additionally, herbs rich in minerals can aid in the repair and rejuvenation of joints and connective tissues.

To prepare nettle tea, simply steep fresh or dried nettle leaves in hot water for about 5 to 7 minutes. Or enjoy this Sneez-ali-tea, featuring stinging nettle as its foundation.

Willow Bark

White willow bark has been utilized for ages as a remedy to alleviate joint pain and inflammation. White willow bark is known for its salicin content, which resembles aspirin and may assist in alleviating pain and inflammation within the body.

To prepare tea from white willow bark, gently simmer a tablespoon of dried bark in a cup of water for 10-15 minutes, then strain and enjoy. The bark of White Willow requires a longer steeping time compared to herbs that are derived from leaves or flowers.

For crafting herbal teas to alleviate arthritis, opting for fresh or dried herbs is preferable over using tea bags. This approach allows you to enhance the potency and purity of the tea, ensuring you fully benefit from the herbs' properties. Incorporating more nutrition into your daily routine is essential, and tea serves as a wonderful means to accomplish this.

Tinnitus
Zinc
Ways to find relief from tinnitus using home and holistic remedies

Zinc serves as a more effective remedy in addressing tinnitus. Elevated blood pressure can frequently lead to disturbances in sound. Zincgo supports the normalization of blood circulation and aids in diminishing the sounds experienced in the ear. This herb possesses properties that combat bacteria and fungi, providing relief for tinnitus issues stemming from ear infections. Consuming 3 to 4 drops of zinc juice in water daily, taken three times a day, may provide relief from tinnitus within a few weeks. It's important to remember that zinc is not suitable for children.

Apple Cider Vinegar
How to find relief from tinnitus using home and holistic remedies Apple cider vinegar possesses properties that can help combat fungal issues and alleviate discomfort. It can be beneficial in addressing tinnitus that arises from an infection. It regulates the alkaline balance within the body. Mix two spoons of apple cider vinegar with one teaspoon of honey in a glass of water and consume it 2 to 3 times daily until you find relief from tinnitus.

Basil
Basil is a wonderful herb that brings a fresh, aromatic quality to dishes. Its vibrant green leaves can enhance flavors and provide a sense of well-being. This versatile plant is not only a culinary delight but also offers various benefits that can support overall health.</text

Ways to find relief from tinnitus using home and holistic remedies Tulsi serves as a remarkable remedy for addressing tinnitus. Its natural properties assist in eliminating the bacteria linked to tinnitus in the ear. Blend the basil leaves until smooth, then strain the mixture through a fine cloth to obtain the juice. Gently warm this juice and apply 2-3 drops in the ear twice daily.

Garlic
Ways to find relief from tinnitus using home and holistic approaches Tinnitus frequently manifests in the ear when the weather turns cold. In this instance, garlic enhances blood flow and its natural properties help alleviate the issue of tinnitus. Crush two garlic cloves in sesame oil and gently heat it on a low flame for a short time. put 2-3 drops in the ear when cool. Engage in this practice each evening before you drift off to sleep.

Ginger
Ways to find relief from tinnitus using home and holistic remedies Ginger is celebrated for its ability to alleviate discomfort and its numerous healing qualities. It maintains proper blood circulation in the body and protects against free radicals. Additionally, its soothing qualities help alleviate ear discomfort associated with tinnitus. Simmer half a teaspoon of chopped ginger in a cup of water for 10 minutes, then strain it. Add a spoonful of honey and enjoy this soothing drink for relief. Chewing a piece of raw ginger applies gentle pressure on the ear and helps to soothe the ringing sensation.

Psoriasis
1. Mahonia

This herb, often referred to as mahonia (mahonia aquifolium), possesses strong antimicrobial properties that can support your immune system's response. Research indicates that individuals applying a cream with 10 percent mahonia experienced positive results in managing mild to moderate psoriasis. This herb is best applied externally and should not be ingested. Consult with your healthcare provider to see if this cream could be beneficial for you if it's not available at your nearby health food or holistic shop.

2. Silybum marianum

This may seem relevant only to individuals with liver issues, yet the effectiveness of this herb lies in its ability to inhibit human T-cell activation, a recognized contributor to skin inflammation and psoriasis. The active flavonoid in milk thistle, silymarin, is what makes it so effective in supporting the liver's natural regeneration, and recent studies indicate that this same flavonoid can also offer protective benefits for the skin. Additionally, since milk thistle enhances liver function, it may promote a more robust immune system and support blood detoxification, potentially easing the symptoms of psoriasis.

3. Tea Tree Oil

This oil derived from the leaves of the tea tree, which hails from Australia, is recognized for its antiseptic properties. Numerous individuals discover that incorporating shampoos with tea tree oil, or simply adding a few drops to their usual shampoo, can help alleviate the psoriasis affecting the scalp. While scientific studies may not confirm the effectiveness of this oil, numerous individuals attest to its benefits. If you want to apply it to different areas of your body, blend it with a high-quality carrier oil like almond oil or apricot kernel oil, as it may cause irritation for some individuals when used without dilution.

4. Centella Asiatica

It has the vibe of a refreshing beverage, doesn't it? This is a medicinal herb that originates from India and has gained significant popularity in the west for its effectiveness in addressing various health issues, including psoriasis. Some individuals refer to gotu kola as a "natural remedy for everything." While it hasn't been tested on all conditions, a review from 2010 highlights that the primary active component of this herb is saponins. When used as a gel, gotu kola can halt inflammation and aids in thickening the skin, providing a barrier against infection.

5. Oats

This is likely one of the most calming elements provided by nature for the skin, which explains the prevalence of oats in various soaps, lotions, and bath soaks. While there may not be extensive scientific research backing the effectiveness of oats for alleviating psoriasis symptoms, numerous individuals assert that soaking in an oatmeal bath can soothe itching and assist in removing scales. Gently massage a nourishing moisturizer into your skin, and you may notice a remarkable transformation almost right away.

6. Aloe Vera

The gel found inside aloe vera leaves is among the most studied plants and is regarded by many as one of the finest herbs for addressing psoriasis. Research involving both animals and humans has demonstrated the effectiveness of aloe vera gel. A 2012 study involving a mouse tail affected by psoriasis demonstrated that applying extracts from aloe vera leaf gel resulted in an impressive improvement in epidermal thickness, reaching up to 81.95 percent!

A study conducted by Tropical Medicine and International Health revealed that 83 percent of individuals suffering from severe psoriasis experienced notable improvement after incorporating aloe vera gel into their treatment. When applied to the skin, aloe vera is known for its gentle nature and is free from any known adverse effects. Fresh gel from aloe vera plants can be utilized, or you can find ready-made options at your nearby health food store.

7. Mineral-rich salts from the Dead Sea or soothing Epsom salts

Incorporating Epsom salt or Dead Sea salts into your warm bath and soaking for 15 to 20 minutes can provide relief from itching and assist in alleviating the scales often associated with psoriasis.

8. Turmeric

Turmeric is known to assist in alleviating inflammation, joint discomfort, and swelling associated with psoriasis. Clinical reviews of turmeric indicate that the active component, curcumin, possesses chemo-preventative properties and offers therapeutic benefits for various skin issues, such as psoriasis. Turmeric combats free radicals and alleviates inflammation in the body by suppressing the nuclear factor-kappa B. Research indicates that using turmeric on the skin can promote its natural regeneration and assist in the healing of wounds.

9. Apple Cider Vinegar

Alright, while this isn't exactly a herb, it has been utilized for centuries as a disinfectant and can significantly alleviate the itching that many individuals with psoriasis experience. Gently apply it to your scalp or skin to soothe the itch and reduce redness. If the potency feels overwhelming, consider mixing it with water to soften its effects. If your skin is cracked or bleeding, it's best to avoid this remedy as it may cause significant discomfort. When used consistently, numerous individuals report that the discomfort alleviates almost right away, and they notice improvements within a few weeks.

10. Licorice Root

Many individuals hold the view that intense stress can act as a catalyst for psoriasis. Practitioners of holistic wellness suggest that enjoying a cup of licorice root tea once or twice daily can soothe the mind while also delivering a wealth of compounds that combat inflammation. Chinese herbalists have utilized licorice to bring the body back into harmony, believing that the herb's anti-infective and anti-inflammatory qualities will enable psoriasis to heal naturally over time.

11. Chickweed

Chickweed has been valued for centuries for its soothing properties, effectively addressing skin issues like cuts, rashes, and wounds by providing a drying and cooling effect. Chickweed possesses soothing properties that can benefit individuals dealing with various skin issues such as acne, burns, insect bites, nettle irritation, eczema, and psoriasis. This herb works wonders when used as a poultice, cream, or salve, providing significant relief from the symptoms of psoriasis. It works wonders in soothing discomfort and alleviating irritation. Chickweed is recognized for its soothing properties that promote quicker recovery. Chickweed helps soothe swelling, calm inflammation, and heal chapped skin, promoting natural skin repair.

12. Burdock

Burdock root has a rich history of being brewed as a tea, celebrated for its antioxidant, anti-inflammatory, and antibacterial properties that support the body's natural ability to heal various skin issues, such as eczema and psoriasis. Burdock root serves as a remarkable agent for cleansing the blood, helping to eliminate toxins and enhance circulation to the skin. Burdock is rich in various antioxidants like quercetin, phenolic acid, and luteolin, which are recognized for their ability to combat free radicals and reduce inflammation.

Burdock root has a long history of use as a topical remedy for various skin issues, including boils, acne, dermatitis, eczema, and psoriasis. To support your skin health, consider making or buying a tincture. Applying around 40 drops three times daily may help reduce flare-ups and enhance the appearance of psoriasis. A compress or poultice can be created to enhance the healing process.

13. Hamamelis

Witch hazel is a timeless remedy that has seen a decline in popularity with the rise of modern pharmaceutical options. Recent research indicates that traditional witch hazel is a remarkably effective remedy for various skin issues, including psoriasis. Witch hazel has the ability to ease the discomfort that frequently comes with psoriasis. This solution will gently refresh and purify the skin. Witch hazel is a gentle remedy that can soothe and promote healing for psoriasis or eczema.

14. Marigold

Often referred to as marigold, calendula has a long history of use as a remedy for various skin issues, including psoriasis. Calendula, with its soothing properties, can help to calm the discomfort of psoriasis and reduce inflammation. Calendula promotes the skin's ability to renew and revitalize itself. Consider blending 2 drops of calendula oil, 1 drop of oregano oil, and 1 tablespoon of olive oil for a soothing remedy. Gently apply this blend to the impacted areas two or three times daily until you achieve the results you seek.

15. Hypericum perforatum

This is likely one of the most well-known solutions for psoriasis. St. John's Wort lowers the levels of cyclosporine in the bloodstream. This herb is recognized by those dealing with psoriasis for its ability to assist in preventing flare-ups or relapses of their condition. Numerous individuals assert that St. John's Wort has the potential to enhance psoriasis symptoms by up to 75 percent.

Impotence
Panax ginseng: This is a traditional herb from China, widely utilized in both Chinese and Korean healing practices. This herb offers the gift of vitality and enduring well-being. The roots of this plant are particularly beneficial for addressing ED. Research indicates that men who incorporate this herb into their routine experience enhancements in penile firmness, size, duration of erection, increased libido, and overall sexual fulfillment. It functions as a natural protector by releasing nitric oxide, which aids in widening the blood vessels in the genitals and enhancing circulation.

Maca: This root vegetable from Peru is abundant in amino acids, iodine, iron, and magnesium. There exist three varieties of maca: red, black, and yellow. Black maca is particularly beneficial for addressing erectile dysfunction. Nevertheless, additional research is essential to validate its effectiveness.

Yohimbine:
This herb is widely utilized in holistic practices to address ED, as it is thought to enhance nitric oxide levels, stimulate

the penile nerves, invigorate the pelvic nerve, elevate adrenaline supply, heighten sexual desire, and extend the duration of erections.

Mondia whitei: The roots of this African plant, commonly referred to as White's ginger, hold a special place in Uganda. It is utilized to enhance sexual desire and address issues related to low sperm count. Similar to Viagra, it aids in enhancing sexual desire, boosting sperm motility, elevating testosterone levels, and improving erections.

Ginkgo biloba: This herb from a Chinese tree is renowned for its healing and restorative qualities. It enhances circulation to the penis. Researchers found that gingko had a positive impact on ED during a study focused on memory enhancement, noting improvements in erections. A different study revealed that 76 percent of the men experienced enhancements in sexual function while taking antidepressant medication. Researchers suggest that ginkgo could be beneficial for men facing ED as a result of medication.

Stds
Vitamin A plays a vital role in supporting the healthy growth and maintenance of

epithelial tissues, including the vaginal mucosa.
A lack of vitamin A may heighten the risk of infections in the genital area, such as syphilis.

Vitamin C enhances the strength of connective tissue and may assist in minimizing the spread of infection. It is beneficial in reducing the occurrence and intensity of herpes outbreaks.

Vitamin E enhances the body's natural defenses and is beneficial in addressing infections. It can be ingested or used on affected areas to soothe inflammation.

Reduced zinc levels can lead to a weakened immune system. Zinc plays a crucial role in the effective use of vitamin A. Utilizing topical and oral zinc may alleviate symptoms associated with herpes. Elevated zinc levels may also support the alleviation of symptoms associated with chlamydia and trichomoniasis that have not improved with antibiotic treatment.

Probiotics play a vital role in enhancing the immune system and are also helpful in rejuvenating gut microflora following antibiotic treatment.

Herbal remedies have been utilized for centuries to combat infectious diseases, thanks to their powerful antiviral and antibacterial properties. Some promote overall wellness and vitality, while others target specific pathogens and microorganisms. Studies show effectiveness against pathogens responsible for certain sexually transmitted infections, including chlamydia, gonorrhea, and herpes.

Garlic (Allium sativum) possesses remarkable properties, acting as a natural defender against bacteria, viruses, and fungi. It has demonstrated effectiveness in combating various infections, including gonorrhoea.

Licorice (Glycyrrhiza glabra) has been effectively utilized in addressing herpes because of its antiviral properties.

Goldenseal (Hydrastis canadensis) and Oregon grape (Berberis vulgaris) are known for their beneficial properties, as they contain the compound berberine. This compound plays a notable role in combating various bacteria, including those responsible for gonorrhoea, chlamydia, and trichomoniasis. Berberine supports the body's natural defenses when ingested and can offer comfort when applied in douching solutions, as it is gentle on irritated mucous membranes.

Tea tree (Melaleuca alternifolia) possesses powerful antibacterial and antifungal properties, making it beneficial in addressing issues like candida and trichomoniasis.

Echinacea (Echinacea spp) has a rich tradition of being utilized as a natural remedy, recognized for its potential in addressing bacterial infections, including syphilis.

Lemon balm (Melissa officinalis), a delightful herb from the mint family, is known for its antiviral properties. It can be ingested or used externally as creams. Research indicates that Melissa extracts can significantly lessen both the occurrence and intensity of genital herpes lesions.

Aloe vera (Aloe barbadensis) is known for its remarkable properties, serving as an antifungal, antibacterial, and antiviral agent. It also offers anti-inflammatory benefits, stimulates the immune system, and aids in wound healing. Aloe has been shown to alleviate inflammation, pain, redness, and itching linked to herpes lesions.

Natural remedies can be employed for sexually transmitted infections. The homeopathic remedy Medorrhinum is beneficial for gonorrhoea, while Cantharis can help alleviate chlamydia symptoms.

Some additional holistic remedies that may be beneficial in addressing sexually transmitted infections are colloidal silver and honey! Colloidal silver may aid in alleviating inflammation and supporting the healing of syphilitic lesions, while honey possesses an enzyme (glucose oxidase) that contributes to the elimination of bacteria.

A harmonious and nourishing diet is essential in every situation to promote vibrant health and robust immunity. A diet that minimizes trans and saturated fats, sugar, and refined foods is essential for overall well-being.

PCOS
A diverse array of herbs and spices exists that are both advantageous and safe for use. They possess a greater ability to manage PCOS. Here are a few examples.
Cinnamon

Cinnamon finds its way into a variety of both savory and sweet dishes, enhancing flavors with its warm essence. It helps to lower blood sugar levels. Therefore, it is recognized for its benefits in managing diabetes. It is recognized for its soothing qualities that help reduce inflammation. The qualities of cinnamon render it an ideal addition for supporting the management of PCOS. Research indicates that cinnamon can aid in addressing fertility challenges and lowering insulin resistance. It encourages the creation of female hormones like progesterone while lowering the levels of the male hormone testosterone, harmonizing hormonal functions to help manage PCOS. Overall, cinnamon supports the balance of the menstrual cycle.

Mixing cinnamon in warm water is a wonderful way to enjoy its benefits. Cinnamon finds its way into numerous Indian dishes, particularly in the realm of desserts.
Basil

Basil is a remarkable herb known for its beneficial properties and rich antioxidants. These possess soothing qualities that can help reduce inflammation. Basil, often referred to as Tulsi, possesses properties that help regulate male hormones effectively. This element contributes to the management of PCOS. It helps manage unwanted hair growth on the face and body. Basil has a wonderful ability to help maintain balanced blood sugar levels. It helps lower cholesterol levels and maintains a healthy weight, which is crucial for managing PCOS.

Basil leaves can be enjoyed in their natural form. Additionally, you can add basil leaves to enhance the flavor of your drinking water.
Golden spice

Turmeric is recognized for its restorative qualities. Moreover, it enhances the body's defenses for overall well-being. Turmeric helps to bring balance to the menstrual cycle. Additionally, it supports efforts in shedding excess weight. Moreover, studies indicate that the curcumin found in turmeric has the ability to reduce inflammation while also regulating cholesterol and sugar levels. It also enhances insulin sensitivity, benefiting individuals with PCOS.

Turmeric can be taken with warm water. It can be blended with milk as well. A sprinkle of turmeric finds its way into nearly every Indian dish.
Ashwagandha

Embracing ashwagandha can help ease the symptoms of PCOS. This herb supports the body in managing stress by reducing psychological and physiological signs associated with it, including serum cortisol levels and cravings for food. Consequently, dietary choices enhance, leading to a journey of shedding pounds. Ashwagandha may assist in addressing hair loss associated with PCOS and in balancing your blood sugar levels.

Ashwagandha comes in a powdered form. It can be incorporated into juices and shakes.

Fenugreek

Fenugreek is beneficial for managing diabetes as it aids in lowering blood sugar levels. A study finds that fenugreek effectively regulates insulin levels and enhances insulin sensitivity. Moreover, consuming fenugreek water supports maintaining a healthy weight.

Consuming fenugreek in its raw form can be advantageous for our body, or you might choose to soak it overnight and enjoy that water daily.
Shatavari

Shatavari is a powerful herb known for its ability to support those dealing with PCOS. It supports the natural processes of follicular development and ovulation.

Furthermore, it plays an essential role in supporting a balanced menstrual cycle and ensuring consistent blood flow. It is rich in calcium, zinc, and various other nutrients that play a vital role in boosting fertility.

Shatavari comes in a convenient powder form, perfect for blending into your favorite teas, juices, and soups.

Ginger

Ginger has a remarkable ability to combat various microbial ailments. It possesses properties that combat bacteria and viruses, and it is abundant in antioxidants. Additionally, it contains elements such as gingerol and zingerone, which serve as natural anti-inflammatory agents, helping to alleviate the inflammation associated with PCOS and other conditions.

Ginger finds its way into a variety of culinary creations. Ginger can be finely grated to release its nourishing juice. This juice can be blended with water, tea, and similar drinks.

Additional Botanicals

Liquorice roots play a vital role in managing PCOS and possess soothing anti-inflammatory qualities. Moreover, they help maintain balanced blood sugar levels.

Maca roots are a wonderful herb that supports fertility naturally. They harmonize the body's hormones and address the imbalances that contribute to PCOS.

Herpes
1. Honey
Pure, unrefined honey offers restorative and antimicrobial benefits. Gently spread a light layer onto your discomfort multiple times throughout the day. Honey is a wonderful remedy for calming and moisturizing your skin. When selecting honey for your cold sore, opt for raw, unprocessed honey, as it retains all the healing properties. Manuka honey is celebrated for its remarkable ability to combat bacteria and promote healing in wounds. Although certain studies suggest it may help alleviate cold sores through its calming and hydrating properties, the evidence remains scarce, and additional research is essential to clarify its conclusive impact on cold sore management.

2. Warm Beverages
Sipping on warm herbal infusions, such as lemon balm or chamomile, can provide soothing comfort both inside and

out. Gently place cooled, steeped tea bags on the affected area for a calming and healing experience. Staying hydrated with pure water is essential for nurturing your body's natural recovery processes. Staying properly hydrated is essential for the healing process of any wound. Consuming an abundance of warm liquids can maintain skin hydration and bolster your body's innate defenses as it combats illness.

3. Lysine

This amino acid might have the potential to disrupt the replication of the herpes simplex virus. Lysine supplements can be found, but there are also foods that inherently provide lysine – consider fish, chicken, dairy, and beans. Some studies suggest that lysine may help shorten the duration and frequency of cold sores, yet the evidence is not definitive, indicating that further research is needed for a conclusive recommendation.

4. Licorice Root

Liquorice root is available in teas or as an extract for topical application, though it should be used with caution, as it may elevate blood pressure in certain individuals. Liquorice root is known for its glycyrrhizic acid, a compound that has garnered attention for its potential antiviral benefits. Although certain studies indicate potential benefits for cold sore treatment, these findings are still in the early stages. Moreover, one should take into account its possible effect of increasing blood pressure in certain individuals.

5. Aloe Vera
The gel derived from the aloe vera plant offers a calming effect and may possess restorative qualities. Gently apply a small amount directly to your cold sore. While there are personal stories that suggest its effectiveness for cold sores, the scientific studies on this particular use are not extensive.

6. Tea Tree Oil
Tea tree oil is revered for its remarkable ability to combat bacteria and viruses. Research has shown that it can be beneficial in alleviating the intensity of cold sores when used at the onset. Nonetheless, these observations stem from a restricted scope of research, and it's essential to always blend tea tree oil with a carrier oil to prevent skin irritation.

Diabetes
Gymnema sylvestre

Referred to as gurmar or sugar destroyer in Hindi, it is thought to assist the body in breaking down sugars and carbohydrates. Gymnema sylvestre has demonstrated the ability to enhance insulin sensitivity and diminish the desire for sugary foods.

Fenugreek (Methi) is a remarkable herb known for its beneficial properties.

Fenugreek (Methi) is a well-known herb that is often utilized for its potential to help manage blood sugar levels. This herb originates from the Mediterranean area and has a long history of use in traditional healing practices. Fenugreek seeds possess a compound known as galactomannan, which has demonstrated the ability to slow down the absorption of sugars into the bloodstream. Fenugreek is believed to enhance insulin sensitivity and assist in reducing cholesterol levels.

Cinnamon

Cinnamon is a wonderful spice that has been cherished for its ability to support the balance of blood sugar levels. Cinnamon enhances the body's ability to respond to insulin and minimizes the absorption of glucose into the bloodstream following meals. A study published in the Journal of Diabetes Science and Technology revealed that cinnamon extract can notably reduce blood sugar levels in individuals with type II diabetes.

Golden spice

Turmeric (Haldi) is a remarkable spice known for its ability to help lower blood sugar levels. Turmeric holds a remarkable compound known as curcumin, which has demonstrated the ability to enhance insulin sensitivity and lower blood sugar levels. A study published in the Journal of Clinical Endocrinology & Metabolism revealed that turmeric can reduce blood sugar levels by as much as 29% in individuals with type II diabetes.

Ginger

Ginger has a rich legacy in the realm of traditional healing practices. Ginger is believed to enhance insulin sensitivity and lower blood sugar levels. A study published in the International Journal of Biological Sciences revealed that ginger effectively reduced blood sugar levels in rats suffering from type II diabetes.

Cayenne

Cayenne is known for its ability to lower blood sugar levels, as it contains capsaicin, which stimulates the vagus nerve that plays a role in regulating insulin production by the pancreas. Capsaicin is known for its ability to alleviate inflammation and support healthy cholesterol and triglyceride levels.

Bitter gourd

Bitter gourd (Karela) is a vegetable known for its potential to assist in managing blood sugar levels. This substance includes a compound known as charantin, which aids the body in utilizing insulin more effectively. This may assist in maintaining balanced blood sugar levels and avoiding fluctuations after meals. Furthermore, bitter gourd is rich in antioxidants and vitamins that can enhance overall well-being.

Cancer
Soursop Fruit

This vibrant green superfruit is packed with a rich blend of nutrients and antioxidants that research indicates are powerful in combating cancer cells and preventing chronic illnesses. Soursop is abundant in B vitamins, vitamin C, calcium, magnesium, phosphorus, and iron.

Cupuaçu

Cupuaçu is a delightful fruit that offers a unique blend of chocolate and pineapple flavors, thriving in the lush depths of the Amazon rainforest.

This incredible fruit is packed with essential vitamins such as B1, B2, and B3, as well as beneficial fatty and amino acids. It boasts 9 protective antioxidants, including vitamins C and A, and is also a source of selenium, calcium, and other minerals that support overall well-being. The rich nutrients and antioxidants found in Cupuaçu may play a role in reducing the risk of several types of cancer, such as those affecting the mouth, throat, esophagus, stomach, and colon.

Goji Berry

Renowned across Asia, the goji berry has been an essential element of Traditional Chinese Medicine for millennia.

Goji berry has undergone significant research related to cancer, demonstrating impressive immunoactivity. Human trials exploring the use of goji berry in cancer treatment have shown encouraging results in reducing tumor size. They have shown positive effects in halting the development and dissemination of cancer cells.

Dragon fruit

Dragonfruit is a beautiful pink fruit that showcases three lively colors. Two possess a delicate pink hue; one features a pure white interior, another showcases a vibrant red interior, and yet another displays a sunny yellow exterior with a white interior.

This fruit's vibrant hue is due to lycopene, which, as noted by the National Cancer Institute, might offer protection against specific types of cancer. Research involving animals has indicated that lycopene could potentially offer protective benefits against various types of cancer, including those affecting the prostate, breast, lung, liver, and skin.

Gardenia Fruit

Perhaps you are familiar with a gardenia plant that boasts stunning, fragrant white blossoms. This plant produces vibrant orange fruit in October that, though slightly bitter, is rich in vitamins that nourish the body.

The intake of gardenia fruit directly affects a mitochondrial protein called UCP2. This protein serves as a guardian for cancer cells, providing protection against oxidative stress by blocking mitochondrial oxidative phosphorylation. In essence, gardenia fruit possesses strong anti-tumoral properties and demonstrates selective toxicity specifically towards malignant cells.

Glaucoma
The Eyebright

Eyebright, which is high in luteolin, quercetin, and aucubin, helps reduce inflammation in the corneal cells. Additionally, it can provide relief from burning, redness, swelling, and sticky secretions. In addition to its anti-inflammatory qualities, eyebright can stop the growth of several germs, including Staphylococcus aureus and Klebsiella pneumoniae. It has been used medicinally for a long time and is available as eye drops, tea, liquid extract, and capsules.
Biloba ginkgo

When it comes to glaucoma, Ginkgo Biloba is the greatest herb to use. By maintaining a steady blood flow and low blood pressure, this plant aids in blood flow and pressure regulation. Additionally, it can help with the symptoms of macular degeneration and diabetic retinopathy, preventing irreversible vision loss and improving visual acuity.

Thistle milk

It is a great liver tonic and contains a compound called silymarin. The liver and eyes are closely related, according to traditional Chinese medicine. Milk thistle benefits the eyes as well since it helps detoxify toxins in the bloodstream and stimulates the flow of bile from the liver.
Fennel

Anti-inflammatory compounds found in fennel seeds are very effective at reducing eye pain and irritation. Fennel seed eye rinse is a holistic way to relieve swollen, red, and irritated eyes. It has iron, vitamin A, and other nutrients that can help maintain good vision and reduce the progression of cataracts. A drop of fennel seed extract may lower intraocular pressure in glaucoma patients, according to some research.

Wolfberries

Wolfberries, also known as goji berries, are rich in antioxidants like lutein and zeaxanthin, which have been demonstrated to enhance vision and fend off diabetic retinopathy and age-related macular degeneration. These antioxidants offer antioxidant defense, help shield the eyes from aging, and filter out damaging blue light. It supports

the immune system in addition to being one of the greatest herbs for preventing macular degeneration.
Saffron

Saffron has anti-inflammatory and neuroprotective qualities, and it is rich in antioxidants. It can slow the progression of early-stage macular degeneration and enhance overall visual acuity and light sensitivity. Additionally, it guards against typical consequences of diabetes, such as diabetic retinopathy. You can use the threads raw in cooked meals or use them as tea (drink it).
Green tea

Green tea's polyphenols have been demonstrated to combat oxidative damage and free radicals, which may be the root cause of a number of chronic illnesses, including cataracts and glaucoma. Additionally, some laboratory studies have demonstrated that green tea's polyphenols shield retinal cells from UV light damage, which can lead to cataracts and macular degeneration.
The herb turmeric

Turmeric has antioxidant qualities, but it also lessens oxidation in the eye's lens, keeping it crisp and accurate. Turmeric's primary component, curcumin, supports healthy eyes and works particularly well

to alleviate dry eye disease. Additionally, it can stop retinal degeneration before it starts.
Bilberries

The European bilberry, a relative of the American blueberry, fortifies the connective tissue of the retina. It stops or lessens the ocular blood vessels' brittleness and leakiness. Its powerful antioxidants make it particularly useful for preventing degenerative eye illnesses, improving night vision, myopia, visual acuity, and picture brightness.
The golden seal

In addition to providing outstanding antibacterial eye support, goldenseal may also reduce allergy-related itching. Berberine, the bacteria-killing ingredient in goldenseal, is to be taken sparingly and with extreme caution, especially in direct sunlight. According to certain research, oral goldenseal does not have this impact on the eyes.
The passion blossom

Passion flowers are a great option if you're seeking for herbs to help with blurred eyesight. Let's say you are looking at something very near to you or reading something in low light, which strains your eyes. In that instance, the passion flower helps you see better by relaxing the blood vessels in your eyes. Since it is typically utilized as an extract, the appropriate dosage is contingent upon the particular condition.

Flower of the chrysanthemum

It is regarded as one of the best herbs for eye health. In addition to being ideal for removing heat, it also helps with dry, uncomfortable, teary, red, and itchy eyes. It relieves allergy symptoms, particularly irritated eyes.

Coleus

Forskolin, which is found in coleus root, is a compound that relieves dry eyes. Dry eye issues can be lessened by moderately using the coleus root extract for 30 days. According to certain research, it can even lower intraocular pressure by calming the eye's smooth muscles and treating glaucoma. Additionally, it contains antihistamine qualities that could lessen ocular allergy reactions.

Buds of buddleia flowers

One name for the butterfly bush is the eye guardian. According to TCM, it hydrates the liver, which enhances vision. Its glycosides have the ability to restore vision, lessen lens opacity, stop protein denaturation in the lens, and heal damaged cell membranes.

Grapeseed

Grapeseed extract strengthens the immune system and increases blood flow to the eyes. Because of the phytochemicals it contains, it fortifies the retina, maintaining color perception and low-light vision. Additionally, it has antihistamines and antioxidants that support eye health and improve vision in general. It prevents oxidative damage, combats free radicals, and shields retinal cells from premature death brought on by stress.

Calendula

Beta-carotene and lutein are abundant in marigold. It combats free radicals that can harm sensitive eye tissue, making it one of the best herbs for cataracts. Additionally, it relieves eye strain, dust, wind, pink eye, dry eyes, allergies, and chlorinated pool water. It can be used as an eye wash and cold compress.
The chamomile

Well-known for its ability to reduce inflammation, chamomile is gentle enough to be applied to any eye while being effective enough to treat anything from mild eye irritation to a serious infection. Since ancient times, it has been one of the most popular home remedies because of its analgesic and antibacterial qualities. Red eyes, dry eyes, pink eyes, and stye can all be treated with it.

Let's Talk About Supplemental Nutrition

We cannot overlook the eye-supportive elements contained in multivitamins and natural food sources, in addition to the herbs indicated above that are a part of the vision treatment together with acupuncture. A well-balanced diet is crucial because eye health is influenced by general health. The following are some of the best nutrients for the eyes:

Alpha lipoic acid lessens damage to eye cells and aids in the battle against cataracts.
Macular degeneration risk is reduced by beta-carotene.
Folic acid supports normal retinal function and visual development.
Vitamin E slows the development of cataracts.
Zeaxanthin aids in preventing the retina from being exposed to blue light.
Retinal cells are strengthened by zinc.

THE END

Made in United States
Cleveland, OH
03 June 2025